Pregnancy Tips

for

The Clueless Chick™

Sourced Media Books, LLC
20 Via Cristobal
San Clemente, CA 92673
www.sourcedmediabooks.com

ISBN-13: 978-1-937458-47-8
LCCN: 2012910462

Printed in the United States of America.

This publication is designed to provide entertainment value and is sold with the understanding that the publisher is not engaged in rendering legal, accounting, or other professional advice of any kind. If legal advice or other expert assistance is required, the services of a competent professional person should be sought.

—From a Declaration of Principles jointly adopted by a Committee of the American Bar Association and a Committee of Publishers and Associations

Pregnancy Tips

for

The Clueless Chick™

Jennifer Durbin

Sourced Media Books, LLC
San Clemente, CA

To my little guys and my big guy.

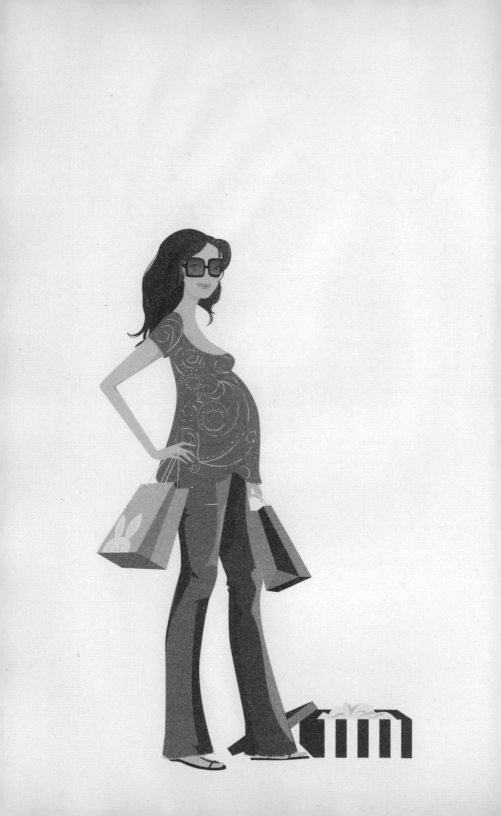

Contents

Foreword

*P*regnancy Tips for The Clueless Chick™ is the first pocket guide for the professional woman who would spend hours reading pregnancy books and reviewing websites, if she had more than five minutes to spare in her busy day. Written by the quintessential Type-A/OCD overachiever, The Clueless Chick™ is a collection of pocket guides for navigating through the milestones and obstacles all women, girlfriends, wives, and mothers face. First and foremost, I'm not a medical expert, and I'm not professionally trained in the areas I discuss in my books. What I am is a woman just like you, albeit a little obsessed with overresearching life's little challenges; and I'd like to share what I've learned from my experience. My hope is that I will be able to save you hours of research and days of searching hundreds of websites in your quest for the one kernel of knowledge you are looking for. *Pregnancy Tips for The Clueless Chick™* will afford you the time to focus on what is fun about being pregnant: spending time with your partner, shopping, picking out baby names, and enjoying every little kick and jab. When you are finished with this pocket guide, you will feel less "clueless"—armed with a roadmap to lead you through this adventure you are embarking on.

Pregnancy Tips for The Clueless Chick™ is a compilation of everything I wish I had known during my first and second pregnancies. Yes, there are in fact lots of new things you learn each pregnancy. You can think of this as a pregnancy quick-start guide based upon all of the research I have done. My pregnancy advice comes straight from my experiences, the experiences of my girlfriends, and the countless books, websites, pamphlets, and research papers I have scoured trying to find the answer to every question I had. If you are pregnant, or just trying, and feel completely clueless, I am here to clue you in!

Whether this is your first or your third pregnancy, this pocket guide will give you the tips and tricks you need to survive the next 40 weeks and prepare for the craziness that is parenthood. This book will not answer all of your medical questions, nor will it tell you what to do. This book is intended to help you make informed decisions—and believe me, the number of decisions facing pregnant women today can be overwhelming. Being pregnant can be a wonderful experience; and the more informed you are, the better your journey will be. Ultimately, my goal for this book is to spare you and other women the tremendous frustration that comes with being completely clueless about pregnancy. Advice can be wonderful, but you've got your own brain—so use it!

You will be making more decisions than you ever thought possible over the coming ten months. Yes, do the math . . . 40 weeks is *much* longer than nine months! So buckle up and enjoy the ride!

There are two terms I use throughout this book that deserve a bit of clarification. We all arrive at this stage in our lives from different points—every woman, pregnancy, and baby is uniquely wonderful. I often refer to your "partner." This may be your husband, the father of your child, your partner, or simply the sister or good friend who will be there to support you throughout your pregnancy and, most importantly, be there to hold your hand in the delivery room. I will also refer to your "doctor." This may be your OB/GYN, midwife, doula, or other health care provider you have chosen to rely on for medical advice.

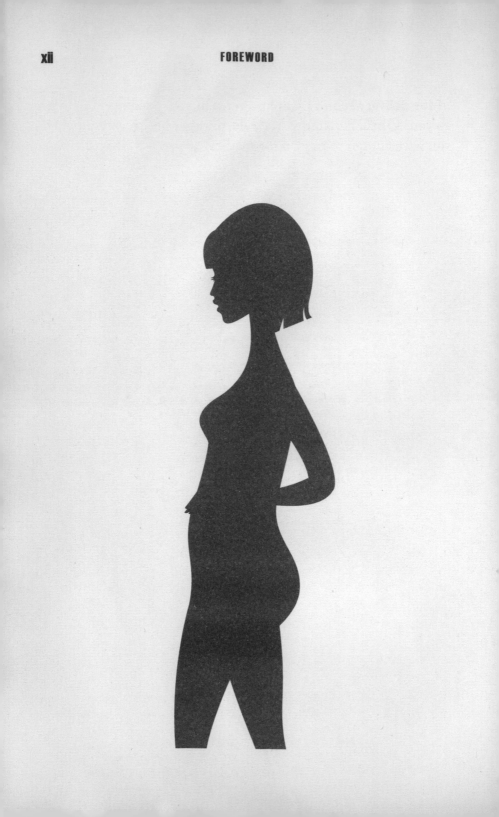

The First Trimester

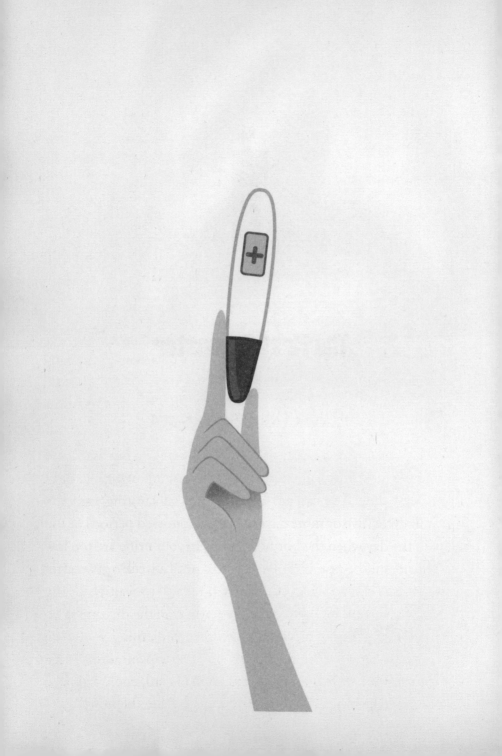

1

What to Do When
You Think You're Pregnant

Congratulations! Whether you have been trying to conceive for years or simply forgot to take your pills, here are the top three things you'll need to do first.

1. Take a Home Pregnancy Test

If you suspect that you may be pregnant, go out and buy a home pregnancy test. You will probably want to invest in a pack of at least three. You can get a false negative by testing too early in your cycle (five or more days before your missed period) or too late in the day when the hormone levels in your urine are too low to register on the test. It is safest to wait until a week or two after your missed period. Yes, yes, I know it is hard to wait that long (at least it was for me!). Most importantly, read the directions on the package. If you are considering doing something special to surprise your partner with the exciting news, plan accordingly. You may want to buy a "Congratulations!" card, cook a special dinner, or take him to your favorite spot to share the news.

2. Visit Your Doctor

As soon as you have positive confirmation from your home pregnancy test, call your doctor to make an appointment. If it is still very early in your pregnancy, your doctor may draw blood to perform a more conclusive pregnancy test. Your first Obstetrical (OB) appointment may be with a nurse where you will simply discuss your medical history and decide on which prenatal tests you may or may not elect to have performed; or you may meet with your doctor to have an ultrasound during which they will determine how far along you are (i.e., your gestational week). This is when they will set your official due date! Either way, this is just the first of what will feel like an endless cycle of appointments by the time you reach 40 weeks. You will also likely discuss your insurance coverage and possibly work out a co-pay payment plan.

If you have not already selected a doctor, this is the time to start looking! If there is a hospital or birth center in your area where you and your partner would like to deliver, you can contact them to get a list of affiliated doctors. Don't be afraid to get recommendations from friends, coworkers, neighbors, or the pregnant lady in line in front of you at the grocery store. You can always tell them that you are starting the planning process early or asking on behalf of a "friend."

Once you have narrowed your list down to two or three doctors, schedule a meet-and-greet appointment with each of them. Most doctors are happy to take the time to meet with you and your partner. This initial meeting will give you an opportunity to discuss what is important to you and ensure that you and your doctor are a good fit. It is extremely important that you agree on the same general philosophies. For instance, if you are open to the use of an epidural or other pain medications during delivery, you don't want to select a doctor who is opposed to the use of any pain medication. It is also a good idea to include your partner if he will be playing an active role in your pregnancy.

Questions to Ask a Prospective Doctor

Here are a few basic questions you can ask a prospective doctor (a 15-minute online search will give you additional ideas). Just remember to keep the number of questions to a reasonable length. You don't need to show up with five pages of questions:

Insurance and Billing

❑ Do you accept my insurance?

❑ Will you prepare a payment plan for me?

The Practice

❑ How many doctors are in your practice? Will I meet with each doctor in your practice?

❑ How long have you been in practice?

❑ Are you board certified?

❑ Will you deliver my baby, or will it be the doctor who is on call that day?

❑ Can I speak directly to you if I have questions in between appointments?

❑ If my pregnancy is deemed "high risk," will I continue to see you, or will you refer me to another practice?

❑ Will I have to go to a lab each time blood must be drawn, or do you have a facility onsite?

❑ How frequently will I have prenatal appointments?

❑ Will there be time for me to ask questions during my appointments?

❑ Do you offer childbirth classes?

Delivery

❑ What hospitals and birth centers are you affiliated with?

❑ Will you support my birth plan and medication preferences?

❑ Will you support my decision to involve a midwife or doula in the delivery?

3. Decide Whom to Tell and When

Being pregnant is an exciting time, and it is exciting news you'll want to share with friends, family, and coworkers. Many women share the exciting news with anyone who will listen as soon as they find out, while others are more cautious and choose to wait until the second trimester when they have passed the highest risk period for miscarriage. Waiting to share your news also gives you and your partner time to make decisions about your pregnancy and post-pregnancy plans (will you go back to work, will the baby go to day care, will you be sharing the baby's name before he or she arrives, etc.), and it gives you a brief reprieve from all of the unsolicited pregnancy advice you will receive.

However you handle your pregnancy announcement is truly up to you. My husband and I decided to wait until we made it past the 12-week milestone before we "officially" announced my pregnancies to friends, family, and coworkers. But if truth be told, there were a few very close friends with whom we shared the news immediately. A good rule of thumb if you are going to tell people immediately is that you should only tell the friends and family members whom you would tell about any possible complications. It is also nice to have someone to confide in on those days when your morning sickness is getting the best of you.

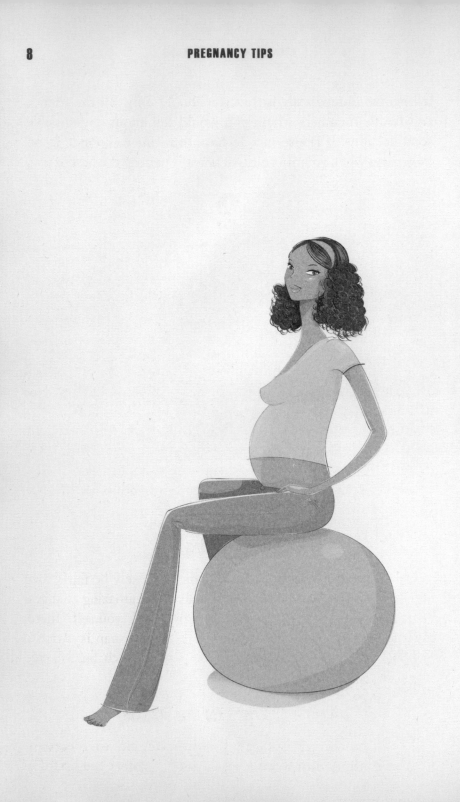

2

Make Your Baby's Health Your #1 Priority

Most of the information in this section should be self-explanatory, but some points may surprise you. It is very important to remember that you now have another life dependent upon your health, and anything harmful you put in your body can and will likely harm your baby. The most important things to remember are to rest, to continue to exercise, and to watch what you eat and drink.

Start Resting

During your first trimester, you will likely be fairly low on energy as your body goes through all of the amazing changes associated with pregnancy—so don't overbook yourself. There may be days or even weeks when an afternoon nap is a must. Your body is very busy growing a little person which, believe me, takes a lot of energy!

Don't Stop Your Exercise Routine

Most doctors will tell you to maintain your current exercise routine, with some adjustments to protect you and the baby. If you are a runner, keep running. Before you start a new exercise routine, first talk to your doctor to ensure it is safe for you. Doing something as simple as taking a walk every day can loosen you up and help to ease some labor pains (it is never too early to start preparing your body for labor).

Exercise Ideas

❑ Walk around your neighborhood in the evening or your office park at lunch.

❑ Walk around your local mall. Most malls open their doors to walkers up to 2 hours before stores open.

❑ Sign up for prenatal exercise classes through your local YMCA, gym, or personal trainer. You can find very enjoyable exercise classes like yoga and water aerobics suitable for pregnant women.

Watch What You Eat and Drink

Your doctor may give you a list of what to eat and what to avoid while you are pregnant. If she does not, find a good reference book or reputable website to refer to. We all know that you should not drink alcohol or eat raw fish, but did you know that most doctors recommend that you avoid cold cuts, hot dogs, and unpasteurized cheese? It is also very important to ensure that you are getting all of the vitamins and minerals your baby needs to develop. Since your nutritional needs are different during pregnancy, many doctors will prescribe or recommend a complete prenatal vitamin for you to take every day. Some doctors will advise you to start taking your prenatal vitamins when you start trying to conceive and continue taking them as long as you are breastfeeding.

Dealing with Morning Sickness

Morning sickness is the worst. Let's start with some straight talk: morning sickness does not just hit you in the morning. It can come in the morning, afternoon, or evening, and it can even hang on all day. My husband would always tell people that my morning sickness was the worst between the hours of 6:00 A.M. and midnight.

Even though a lot of women will tell you how wonderful their pregnancy was and that they never felt even a bit uneasy, that's all a bunch of bologna! Aside from a lucky few, most women experience some degree of morning sickness. It is true that most women experience their morning sickness through week 12, but sometimes it holds on through week 16, or 20, or even 40. Morning sickness is anything but fair; chalk it up as part of the ride. There is also the Old Wives' Tale that the worse your morning sickness is, the easier your delivery will be.

Whether you have a hint of nausea for a few days or full-blown morning sickness for months, there are a few tricks of the trade that can go a long way to making you feel a little better. Believe me, every little bit counts!

Tips and Tricks for Surviving Morning Sickness

❑ Drink more water than you thought was even possible, and try to only drink water. You can also try flavored water when you get tired of plain water.

❑ Take your prenatal vitamins right before bed so they don't upset your stomach.

❑ Leave a small bottle of antacids by your bed for when you wake up in the middle of the night with heartburn or indigestion.

❑   Have something to eat the *second* you wake up. Keep crackers by the bed, and have a couple before you even put your feet on the floor. Don't be surprised if you need to have a bowl of cereal before your morning shower and a second breakfast when you get to work.

❑   Always carry a snack with you like raisins, a granola bar, or crackers.

❑   Don't go more than 2 hours without a snack. Apparently this is your body's way of beginning to adjust to the two-hour feeding schedule the baby will be on in the first few weeks.

❑   Don't underestimate how much you may need to eat. At times it will seem like your stomach is a bottomless pit.

❑   Identify your comfort foods and stock up on them.

❑   Suck on a piece of hard candy or a cough drop to help with the nausea and sore throats that can come from heartburn and acid reflux.

❑   Get plenty of sleep. There may even be days when you need a nap or two.

❑   Give motion/sea sickness wristbands a try. It seems a bit odd, but it can help.

❑   When you are feeling up to it, find a prenatal yoga class in your area. The relaxation time will make you feel better and can help with your delivery.

Time to Start Reading

You could go the old-fashioned route, but I would recommend reading something other than the pregnancy book your mother read. I really benefited from having a pregnancy reference guide that walked me through each week of my pregnancies. Don't underestimate how much things will change from one week to the next!

When you are looking at pregnancy books, don't get overwhelmed by their size. You probably won't read them cover-to-cover because there will be chapters that do not apply to your pregnancy. If you read a couple of pages every night, you will be well prepared for what lies ahead (or you will at least have a name for that terrible aching in your hip). The most comforting aspect of reading a pregnancy book is that you will find that most of your symptoms are *very* normal, and reading about them as they are happening will save you a lot of stress and worry—and unnecessary trips to see your doctor. I always found that it was helpful to read a week ahead so that I knew what I was in for in the coming days. As you are reading through your book, jot down any symptoms you are having that are not typical for the week you are in, so that you can ask your doctor about them during your next visits. Most books are very good about explaining all of the most common aches, pains, and funny feelings you will have; but you may be one of the lucky few (like me) who will experience some of the less common symptoms.

Most importantly, *think beyond the book*. Advice is wonderful, but you have to follow your gut! Every pregnancy is different, so don't be surprised if yours is not by the book. And never, ever, ever ignore your own intuition. If you feel that something is wrong or needs to be looked at by your doctor, call her. That is what she is there for.

Recommended Pregnancy Guides

❑   *Mayo Clinic Guide to a Healthy Pregnancy*, by Mayo Clinic

❑   *What to Expect When You're Expecting*, by Heidi Murkoff and Sharon Mazel

❑ *Your Pregnancy, Week by Week* (*Your Pregnancy* Series), by Glade B. Curtis

In addition to a good general pregnancy guide, there are other supplemental books you may want to read (like this one). If you are having multiples, you should consider a supplemental book on carrying multiples. If you are diabetic, you should look for a supplemental book on diabetes and pregnancy, etc. The good news? Not all pregnancy books are dry medical references. You can also choose from a slew of fun pregnancy books. Pregnancy books range from medical reference books to baby product reviews to what Daddy needs to know to survive this wild ride.

Pregnancy and Baby Product Reviews

❑ *Baby Bargains, 8th Edition: Secrets to Saving 20% to 50% on Baby Furniture, Gear, Clothes, Toys, Maternity Wear, and Much More!* by Denise Fields

❑ http://www.babygizmo.com. A great website with product reviews, coupons, and news.

Fun Pregnancy Books

❑ *The Girlfriends' Guide to Pregnancy*, by Vicki Lovine

❑ *Belly Laughs: The Naked Truth about Pregnancy and Childbirth*, by Jenny McCarthy

Don't Forget Daddy

❑ *The Everything Father-To-Be Book: A Survival Guide for Men*, by Kevin Nelson

❑ *The Expectant Father: Facts, Tips and Advice for Dads-to-Be*, by Armin A. Brott

❑ *My Boys Can Swim!: The Official Guy's Guide to Pregnancy*, by Ian Davis

Pregnancy Journals

While 40 weeks may seem like a lifetime at the moment, it will fly by in the blink of an eye. It is fun to keep a pregnancy journal so that you can look back and see exactly what you were going through every step of the way. I even found myself reading my pregnancy journal to reminisce while I was still pregnant!

❏   *The Belly Book: A Nine-Month Journal for You and Your Growing Belly,* by Amy Krouse Rosenthal

Planning Resources

It is simply amazing how many pregnancy planning resources you can find online these days, but which ones are best? In an effort to save you hours of searching, I'd like to share a few of my favorites:

www.justmommies.com/pregnancy_calendar.php. This website offers a fabulous day-by-day pregnancy calendar that can be copied into a spreadsheet to keep track of how the baby is changing every day. It contains fun facts like, "Baby has developed a hand grip reflex," and other interesting tidbits.

www.thebump.com. For those of you who planned your wedding with The Knot, you can now plan your pregnancy with The Bump! The site contains great pregnancy resources and chat rooms.

www.babyzone.com. This website offers lots of pregnancy planning information. You can also sign up for weekly pregnancy update emails, just in case you are having a hard time keeping up with your pregnancy guide reading.

www.babycenter.com. This website also provides great pregnancy planning information and helps you keep track of how big the baby is.

expectnet.com. On this website, you can set up a free online baby pool for friends and family to guess the sex of the baby, birth date, etc.

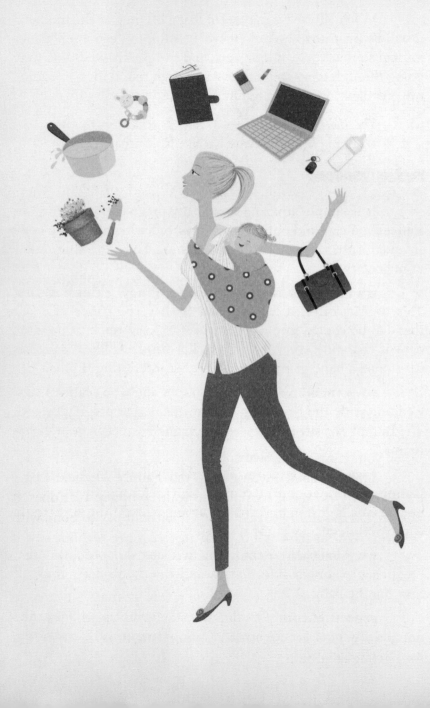

3

Maternity Leave...
Then Back to Work!

Believe it or not, it is never too early to start planning your maternity leave. You'll want to have the details worked out in your mind before you talk to your boss, and you will need to know when to line up childcare if you plan to return to work.

Maternity Leave

All companies handle maternity leave differently, so check with your boss or HR department. You should also read up on your company's leave policies.

I recommend investigating the Family Medical Leave Act (FMLA) to see if it applies to your company. If it does, it affords you the ability to take time off without pay to bond with the baby. Although it is not ideal to take time without pay, it does guarantee that you will have a job when you return to work.

Many employers also offer short-term disability benefits in lieu of maternity leave. The catch here is that you have to enroll in your company's short-term disability plan *before* you get pregnant; once you become pregnant, it is considered a preexisting condition.

When you decide to tell your employer that you are expecting, it is helpful if you have already decided whether or not you plan to return to work after your maternity leave. Do keep in mind that your life will change significantly when the baby is born, and you may change your mind. You may also choose to go back to work only part time, or you may even work out a schedule with your boss where you work part time for your first month or two back at work before transitioning back to full time.

One thing you do not want to do is underestimate how taxing your first couple of weeks back at work will be. Not only will you be readjusting to your old work schedule and catching up on what has happened while you were out, you will also be adjusting to your baby's new childcare routine. The doula who taught our childbirth class gave me a great piece of advice: she said that I would be so drained by the end of my first week back at work that I should plan to take Friday off to recoup. She could not have been more correct! The worst thing you can do is run yourself ragged trying to do everything.

Whether you decide to take 6 weeks or 6 months of maternity leave, it is important to budget accordingly. Unless you are fortunate enough to work for a company that will pay you your full salary while you are on leave, you will likely receive only a portion of your salary for a period of time. You will also need to decide how you would like your taxes to be withheld from short-term disability payments, etc.

Finding the Right Childcare for You

Although it may be several months before the little one arrives, it's never too early to start thinking about how you will care for your baby if/when you decide to go back to work. For those women who plan to stay at home with the baby and not go back to work, you can skip to the next section.

For those of you who will be going back to work after your maternity leave, either part time or full time, and will need to pay for childcare, here are your top three options:

Day Care Center

If you are going to send the little one to a day care center, start looking early! My husband and I didn't visit our first center until week 14 of my first pregnancy, and we were already a bit behind, if you can believe that. If possible, I recommend visiting each day care center you are considering during normal business hours so that you will have a true feel for how it operates. Don't get overwhelmed or stressed about asking every possible question; you will likely take another trip to the center before making your final decision. A good day care center manager will be happy to answer your questions over the phone or via email, and most will be happy to put you in touch with a parent whose child currently attends the day care.

How to Start Your Day Care Center Search

❑ Find your state's Department of Health and Human Services website. Information on childcare is usually found within a child development division or bureau. Your state regulates things such as the maximum infant-to-teacher ratios, feeding practices, etc. and regularly inspects each facility.

❑ Ask friends, neighbors and coworkers what day care centers their children go to.

❑ Research your company's flexible spending account benefits. Many employers offer dependant care flexible spending accounts that can be used for childcare expenses.

❑ Some great national day care resources are nrc.uchsc. edu; acf.hhs.gov/programs/ccb/parents; childcareaware.org; www.childcareservices.org; nccic.acf.hhs. gov; and www.acf. hhs gov/programs/ccb/parents.

In-Home Day Care

In-home day care sounds exactly like what it is: childcare provided in a home, rather than a center, by an adult watching one or a number of children. You can find in-home day cares in your area that are licensed by the state and regulated by the same standards by which day care centers are regulated. There are also in-home day cares that are not licensed or regulated because they do not meet certain criteria. For example, your state may allow in-home day cares to operate unregulated if there are fewer than three unrelated children being cared for. In-home day cares are often significantly less expensive than a day care center and may provide more one-on-one attention than your child will receive in a day care center. In-home day care is also a good way to find religion-based care or a more flexible schedule or curriculum.

Nanny/Au Pair

A nanny is person who provides childcare in the comfort of your own home. An au pair provides the same service but also lives in your home. Hiring a nanny can be extra convenient, because you do not have to transport your child to and from day care, and you can ensure that he or she is in the comfort of your own home. A nanny also provides custom one-on-one care for your child.

Choosing a nanny can be tricky if you do not have any previous experience recruiting a day care professional. You want to find someone who will provide the best care for your child, but you also need to find someone you are comfortable with (especially if this person will be living in your home). There are many places where you can find a nanny: you can retain a local agency, place an add online or at a local university, or search online agencies. I recommend interviewing many candidates, checking their references, and performing background checks.

You may also choose to investigate the possibility of sharing a nanny with a friend or neighbor who has a child or children the same age as your own. This can allow you to save additional money and benefit from the social interaction your children will have with their children. Keep in mind that it will be important to handle this as you would any other business deal and ensure that you and the other family see eye-to-eye on key issues and can work together to sort out any differences or complications that arise regarding your children's care or managing the nanny.

When going the route of a nanny, you'll also need to consider the working arrangement: will the nanny be paid hourly (with or without overtime pay) or a monthly salary? Will you provide any medical benefits or paid time off? What is your backup care plan when the nanny is sick or on vacation? What are the tax and employment law implications for you and the nanny? Are there any citizenship considerations to take into account?

National Nanny Search Resources

- ❑ http://www.care.com
- ❑ http://www.nannies4hire.com
- ❑ http://www.enannysource.com/
- ❑ http://www.greataupair.com/

Questions to Ask a Day Care Provider

Before you visit a day care center, call and ask how much it charges; there is no need to fall in love with a center that you cannot afford. Most day care centers charge either by the week or the month. They also usually charge registration/waitlist fees. In-home care providers may charge by the month, week, or even by the day or hour. It is important to compare all charges if you are looking at multiple centers. Don't forget that day care center rates usually decrease as your child gets older and child-to-teacher ratios increase.

Before you begin interviewing nannies or au pairs you will need to determine how much you are comfortable paying and how comparable that is to the going rate in your area.

Questions to Ask a Day Care Provider

Cost

❑ How much do you charge for infant care?

❑ How often do your rates change?

❑ Do your charges decrease as the child gets older?

❑ What is your payment schedule (i.e., monthly, semi-monthly, or weekly)?

❑ What forms of payment do you accept?

❑ Do you charge any type of annual enrollment, materials, or other fees?

❑ Is there a charge to be placed on your waitlist?

Schedule and Availability

❑ Do you have a slot open to begin caring for my child on _____ date?

❑ What are your normal hours?

❑ Do you charge for early drop-offs or late pickups?

❑ Do you offer part-time slots?

❑ Can I drop in unannounced to visit my child?

Supplies/Materials/Food Provided

❑ What supplies am I responsible for, and what do you provide (diapers, wipes, bibs, etc.)?

❑ Do you provide lunch and snacks for the children?

❑ Are the meals nutritious/organic

Teachers/Care Givers

❑ What are the teachers' qualifications?

❑ What is the discipline philosophy/policy?

❑ Do you provide continuing education for your teachers or have them attend continuing education courses?

Other

❑ Do you require proof of immunizations?

❑ What safety measures do you have in place to protect my child?

❑ What is your sick child policy?

❑ Do you allow shoes to be worn in the infant room?

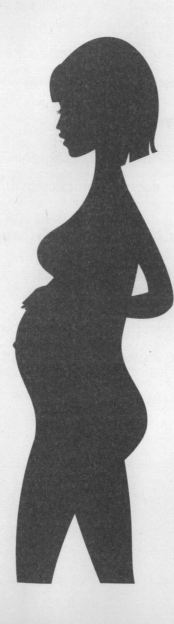

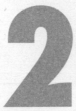

The Second Trimester

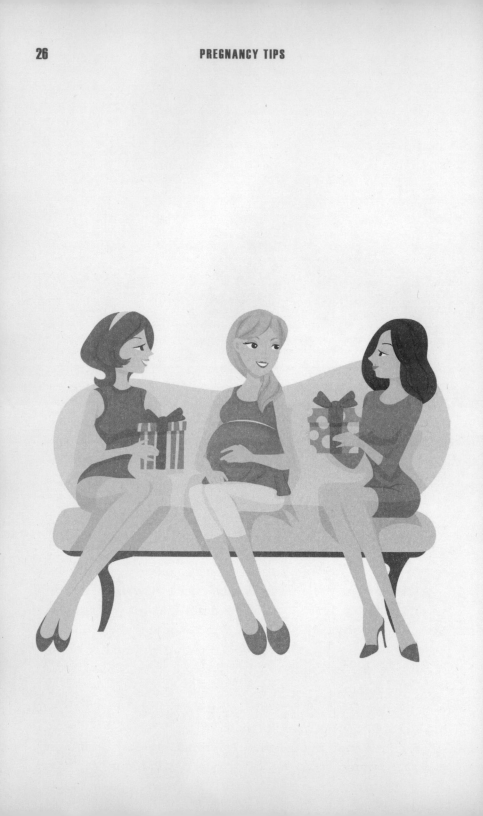

4

Shopping and Showers

Once you enter your second trimester and your belly bump starts to make its appearance, it is time to dive into the fun stuff: shopping and showers! Not only is it time to start shopping for the little one, it is also time to start buying some of those adorable maternity clothes you have been eyeing.

Maternity Clothes

For me, one of the more exciting aspects of being pregnant was getting to buy maternity clothes to show off my baby bump. While shopping can be fun, finding maternity clothes you like within your price range can be tricky. A word of caution: don't buy too much too soon. You never know if you are going to carry the baby high or low, or if you are going to gain weight everywhere or just look like you are carrying around a basketball—all of which greatly impact the type of waistband and fit you will be most comfortable in. I made the mistake of buying too much too early in my first pregnancy, and I wasn't able to wear a number of items I purchased.

You can also take this opportunity to have a little fun with your wardrobe! If you are someone who always purchases the safe, classic pieces, go a little wild and buy something super trendy. After all, whatever you buy is only going to be worn for one season—so have fun with it!

When you start to show and can no longer button your pants (which usually happens around week 12, but we are all different), there are a number of ways to extend the life of your wardrobe.

Tips and Tricks to Extend Your Wardrobe

❑ Loop a rubber band through the front buttonhole on your pants, attaching both ends to the button.

❑ Purchase a Bella Band (http://www.ingridandisabel. com/) or similar product that allows you to leave your pants or skirt unbuttoned and even slightly unzipped.

❑ Zip your skirt halfway and use a safety pin to attach it at the top.

❑ Avoid anything with a defined waist, or switch to wearing only dresses.

There are also a number of ways you can save money on maternity clothes. Consider purchasing key pieces from a consignment store or through Craigslist (http://www.craigslist. org/) or ebay (http://www.ebay.com/). You will find that most maternity clothes you purchase second hand are still in very good condition, because they were not worn very long. Plus, you can benefit from others' mistakes (like mine) of purchasing items too early in their pregnancies that they were never able to wear. You can also borrow clothes from a friend who was recently pregnant. Offer her a free night of babysitting in exchange for taking those maternity clothes that are eating up valuable closet space off her hands for a short time. You can also find alternatives to maternity clothes in the plus section. Just be forewarned that you may not be welcomed with open arms when you stroll into a plus-size store in search of something "big enough to cover your newfound belly."

In addition to the standard maternity stores you will find at the local mall, there are a lot of places you would not think to look for maternity clothes that have some very cute, and often reasonably priced, maternity clothes. While some of these stores offer a good selection of maternity clothes in the store, you will find the largest selection online. Be very mindful of each store's exchange and return policy. Many maternity stores have very strict policies.

Ann Taylor LOFT (http://www.anntaylorloft.com). They currently only offer maternity clothes online. The benefit to shopping here is that you can often find a maternity version of their Misses styles. The downside is that a good portion of what they carry are well-known, high-end brands (not their own) that do not frequently go on sale.

2 Chix (http://www.2chix.com). Not only do they carry very cute and fun graphic T-shirts for you, daddy, and now baby, they carry the most comfortable maternity T-shirts of any place I have found.

Japanese Weekend (http://www.japaneseweekend.com). While their clothes are a bit expensive, they are high-quality, comfortable, and often convertible clothes (from dress to skirt or maternity to nursing). It is worth the investment for the key pieces that you will be wearing frequently or need for the office.

Nordstrom (http://shop.nordstrom.com). You may think that everything at Nordstrom is super expensive, but that is not always the case with their extensive maternity selection. They frequently have sales, and you can get some really great deals on high-end brands.

GAP and Old Navy (http://www.gap.com). Many of the GAP and Old Navy stores carry a selection of maternity clothes in the store, which is very handy. Like the LOFT, you can find maternity versions of their Misses styles so that you don't have to stray far from your own style. They also offer a great selection of casual wear, workout clothes, and sleepwear.

Target (http://www.target.com). Even if you are not someone who usually purchases clothes at Target, check out their maternity section. The quality is good, and the price is right. They also carry very cute maternity bathing suits during the summer and have a great selection of nursing bras and *awesome* nursing camisoles.

Your Local Maternity Boutique. Check your local maternity boutique, even if you are not someone who usually shops in boutiques. You can often find great deals, hard-to-find pieces, and trendy items—or an adorable dress for your shower.

Destination Maternity (A Pea in the Pod, Mimi Maternity, and Motherhood Maternity. http://www.destination-maternity.com). You will always find a sale here and a little bit of everything for every price range. They also carry a good line of nursing clothes.

Baby Showers

Like weddings, babies are a good excuse for your girl-friends, coworkers, or family to throw a shower in your honor. As with any shower, it is a good idea to register for gifts so that your guests know what to get you (and so you don't end up with 20 blankets and no crib sheets).

Registering

While registering is fun, knowing what to register for can be a daunting task if you have never had a child before or don't have an earthly idea of what the difference is between a Baby Bjorn and a Bumbo is (or even what either of them is)!

It is important to keep three things in mind when you are getting ready to register. First, if you are having a baby shower, you will want to complete your registry before the invitations are mailed to accommodate any early shoppers. Second, if you are not having a baby shower, you will still want to register one or two months before your due date. Keep in mind that there will be people who purchase gifts off of your registry after the birth of the baby, so be sure to keep your registry up-to-date. Third, you will also want to ensure that there is a good variety of items still listed on your registry for a coworker with a $15 budget as well as your aunt, who wants to make a *big* impression with her gifts.

These days, there are endless registry options. You can register at a traditional baby superstore, a discount store, an on-line retailer, or your local baby boutique. When you are picking where to register, think about who will be purchasing gifts for you. If your shower guest list includes mostly friends and family who don't know what "amazon.com" is, stay away from online-only registries. If your shower guest list includes everyone from your home town, avoid registering at a baby boutique 30 miles away. One of the main reasons to register is to make the gift-giving process easy on your guests.

There are pros and cons associated with each type of store that offers a baby registry:

Baby Superstore

❑ Pros: Great selection (including diapers, formula, etc.); online registry options.

❑ Cons: Prices can be a bit higher.

Discount Stores

❑ Pros: Great prices; variety of staple items such as diapers, formula, and general household items; online registry options.

❑ Cons: Selection can be limited; return and exchange policies can be stringent.

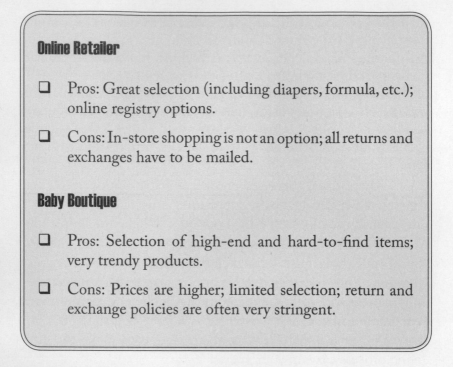

Online Retailer

❏ Pros: Great selection (including diapers, formula, etc.); online registry options.

❏ Cons: In-store shopping is not an option; all returns and exchanges have to be mailed.

Baby Boutique

❏ Pros: Selection of high-end and hard-to-find items; very trendy products.

❏ Cons: Prices are higher; limited selection; return and exchange policies are often very stringent.

What to Do with Everything You Receive

After opening all of your gifts at your baby shower and receiving packages in the mail, it is very tempting to unwrap everything and put it away in the nursery—but not so quick! You will want to unwrap everything that you have to have to bring the baby home (car seat, crib, sleepers, etc.). But you may want to get to know your new buddle of joy a little before you unwrap everything, in case you need to make a few exchanges or returns. For example, you may love the ten different styles of footed sleepers you registered for, but the baby may prefer to sleep in a sleep sack.

On the same note, there are some babies who are very finicky about the types of pacifiers and bottle nipples they will take. If you open and wash all of your bottles at once only to learn two months later that your little one hates the nipples, you will end up shelling out a lot of money purchasing replacements.

Baby Registry Must-Haves

When you are registering, focus on what you will need in the first four to five months. Everything else can wait. You don't want your favorite aunt to spend $150 on a high chair that you won't use until the little one is four months old, when what you *really* need is a swing in the first few weeks. For that reason, you will not see items like high chairs, teething rings, or solid food supplies on my "Must-Haves" list. By registering for items that you do not need for a number of months, you run the risk that you will not receive items you do need immediately. If you find that everything is flying off of your registry, by all means add those items!

While I recommend purchasing all of the items listed below, there are a select few items that you simply cannot live without (e.g., they will not allow you to leave the hospital without a proper infant car seat). Those items are noted in italics below.

When you are deciding between two different brands or styles, don't forget to read customer reviews and check to ensure that a product has not been recalled by the Consumer Product Safety Commission (http://www.cpsc.gov) or a consumer advocacy group, such as Safe Kids (http://www.safekids.org), which will send you recall update emails. You will find that two different brands of baby carriers have extremely different functionality pros and cons. If you want to see how a stroller folds or a baby carrier is worn, play with the items on display in the store or check out www.youtube.com. You would be amazed at the number of product demos and reviews there are on YouTube; in fact, that is how I learned to use my Baby Bjorn and Moby Wrap.

Nursery Furniture

❑   *Crib*
❑   Changing table

- ❑   Dresser
- ❑   Rocker, glider, or recliner
- ❑   Bookshelves
- ❑   Nightlight (check your local home improvement store)

Nursery Miscellaneous

- ❑   Baby clothes hangers
- ❑   Baskets or organizers (for diapers, wipes, toys, etc.)
- ❑   Humidifier or vaporizer
- ❑   Diaper pail (deodorizers, bags, etc.)
- ❑   Small trash can
- ❑   Clothes hamper
- ❑   Ceiling fan (to ensure proper air circulation while the baby sleeps)
- ❑   Safety items (outlet covers, cord hiders, blind cord attachments, etc.)

Clothes

In the first couple of months you will want to dress your baby with one layer more than you are wearing, since they do not produce as much body heat.

- ❑   *Hats*
- ❑   Onesies (short-sleeved and long-sleeved)
- ❑   Pants
- ❑   *Sleepers*
- ❑   One-piece rompers
- ❑   Socks
- ❑   Hand covers (baby mittens or newborn socks)

❑ Seasonal clothes (light sweaters for the fall, heavy clothes for the winter)

❑ Swaddlers or sleep sacks

❑ Going-home outfit (for the trip home from the hospital)

Other Linens

❑ *Hooded towels and washcloths*

❑ *Fitted crib sheets* (2–3). You will also need a waterproof liner if your crib mattress is not waterproof. It saves time and money to find a waterproof mattress for inconvenient messes.

❑ Crib bumper. You can get either a traditional bumper (to protect their little heads from hitting the crib slats), or a breathable bumper (to prevent them from using the bumper as a climber or getting their little faces buried in a padded bumper).

❑ Pack 'n Play sheet (1–2)

❑ Changing pad covers (2–3)

❑ Boppy covers (2)

❑ *Blankets* (for covering the infant carrier when you take the baby out in the first few weeks or for swaddling on the go)

❑ Bibs (for spit up and drool)

❑ *Burp cloths* (small and large)

❑ *Baby laundry detergent* (Dreft or other dye-free and fragrance-free detergent). Most pediatricians will recommend using this throughout the first year.

❑ Nursing cover (for nursing in public or when you have houseguests)

Travel Gear

☐   *Infant car seat*

☐   Diaper bag

☐   Sun shade (or two) for the car

☐   Extra car seat base (if the baby will be riding in more than one car)

☐   Backseat mirror (so you can see your little one while you are driving)

☐   *Stroller frame* (to snap the infant carrier into). This is preferable to a travel system because it is much lighter and more compact. It is easier to get in and out of the car and won't take up the entire trunk!

☐   Jogging stroller (for long hikes or just tooling around the neighborhood)

☐   Baby carrier (Baby Bjorn, ERGObaby, Moby Wrap, sling, etc.)

Play Gear

☐   Swing. Try to find one that plugs in so that you do not burn through batteries.

☐   Bouncy seat/Papasan. This is a mobile and great place for the baby to hang out in the bathroom while you are in the shower.

☐   Crib mobile. Make sure you get a battery-operated one that plays for 10–15 minutes. Some even have remotes.

☐   Play gym. Many come with a baby pillow, which is great for tummy time.

☐   Pack 'n Play. This is a great changing table and nap spot for the living room during the first two months when the baby is going to sleep the majority of the day. If you are short on space, consider the smaller, travel-light version.

Miscellaneous Gear

❑ Itzbeen. This is a must-have! It keeps track of baby's last feeding, which side you last nursed on, the last diaper change, and the last nap. A timer can be set for each. There are also smartphone apps similar to the Itzbeen, such as Baby Brain and Baby ESP.

❑ Boppy (for breastfeeding)

❑ Bumbo

❑ Pacifiers and clips. Get a few different kinds to try. Make sure to get a holder that clips onto baby's clothes.

Bottle-Feeding Gear

You will need bottles even if you are exclusively breastfeeding if you ever want to leave your baby in the care of a friend or relative. The type and number of bottles you buy comes down to personal preference. Most bottles have at least four parts (bottle, nipple, ring, and lid); and some bottles have additional flow regulators or inserts to help minimize gas or colic.

If you are exclusively breastfeeding and will only be using bottles for the occasional supplemental formula feeding or to let Daddy or a caregiver feed the baby expressed breast milk, you will only need one or two bottles. However, if you are bottle feeding your baby every two to three hours, you will probably want at least enough bottles to get you through a 24-hour period. Washing bottles more than once a day, with everything else that is going on, can be very taxing.

You will only need the smaller four-ounce bottles in the beginning; but, by about three months, you will likely move up to the next nipple size and the eight-ounce bottles.

Even if you are planning to exclusively breastfeed, it is good to have at least a little of formula on hand for the few days before your milk comes in, the times you are just too sore to continue nursing, or during those crazy growth spurts. Don't underestimate how much a baby can put away!

❑   Bottles

❑   Bottle brush

❑   Bottle warmer

❑   Pitcher with lid (for making larger quantities of formula if you are exclusively bottle feeding)

❑   Dishwasher basket (for bottle parts, pacifiers, teething rings, spoons, you name it)

❑   Bottle drying rack (because you'll be washing a lot of bottles by hand)

❑   Formula

❑   Powder formula dispenser (for your diaper bag)

Health and Safety Gear

❑   Video monitor. If baby is sleeping outside of your bedroom, or you will be in another room while the baby is sleeping, a monitor is a must. For mommies who worry as much as I do, a video monitor is a must. It will save you numerous needless trips into the nursery to check on the baby—you can simply turn on the video monitor and see what the little one is up to.

❑   Nose bulb

❑   Nail file/nail clippers

❑   *Thermometer and covers*

❑   Baby lotion. This needs to be used very sparingly on newborns, so there is no need to stock up immediately.

❑   Infant saline nasal drops/spray for stuffy noses

❑   *Cotton swabs.* Safety swabs will prevent you from going too deep into the baby's ear, and regular cottonswabs are perfect for cleaning the umbilical cord stump.

❑   *Rubbing alcohol* (for cleaning the umbilical cord)

❑   Vasoline (if you are having a boy who will be circumcised)

❑   Mylicon (in case the little one has gas)
❑   Infant Tylenol
❑   Aquaphor (great for your poor, overwashed hands)

Bathing

❑   Infant bath
❑   *Head-to-toe body wash*
❑   Hairbrush

Diapering

❑   *Diapers.* Buy some newborn diapers, but more size 1—
    the baby will go through eight to ten diapers every day in
    the beginning. Try multiple brands, including store
    brands such as Target. "Blowouts" are a sure sign that you
    need to move up to the next size.
❑   *Wipes,* wipes, and more wipes!
❑   Diaper rash cream
❑   Portable changing pad

Other Must-Haves

❑   Thank you notes (for baby gifts, meals, etc.)
❑   Camera/video camera
❑   Baby book or scrapbook
❑   Hand sanitizer
❑   Antibacterial hand soap in your favorite scent

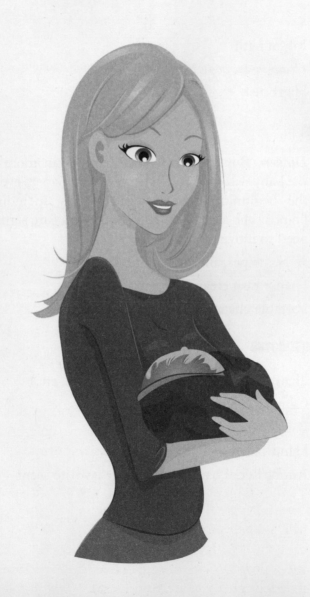

5

Finding the Right
Pediatrician

Finding a pediatrician for your little one before he or she is born is an important and daunting task, if you do not know where to start or what to ask. This is yet another area in which you can benefit from asking for recommendations from friends, coworkers, and neighbors. You may also find that your doctor has a list of recommended pediatricians. You can also get a list of pediatricians affiliated with the hospital or birth center where you will deliver by checking their websites or giving them a quick call.

It is important that you select a pediatrician prior to delivery, because most pediatricians want to see the baby for their first checkup two days after you are discharged from the hospital. During your search, it is also important to keep in mind that if your pediatrician is not affiliated with the hospital at which you will be delivering, she will not be able to admit the baby should complications arise.

Much like your search for a doctor for yourself, it is beneficial to meet with two or three pediatricians to get a better idea of the different styles of care available. It is very important to find a pediatrician you are comfortable with. While you can always change pediatricians, it is important in those first few weeks that you feel comfortable talking to your pediatrician if something is wrong or you have a concern.

Types of Practices

During your search, you will find that your two main options are either a large pediatric practice with a number of doctors, or a small practice with fewer doctors. While each practice is different, you will find that the following holds true:

Large Pediatric Practices

❑ They often offer evening and weekend hours (but charges may be higher).

❑ They may be able to fit in your last-minute appointment, since there are multiple doctors available.

❑ You may not see the same doctor each time.

Small or Private Pediatric Practices

❑ You will see the same doctor each time.

❑ You often receive more personalized care.

Questions to Ask a Prospective Pediatrician

Here are a few basic questions you can ask a prospective pediatrician (a 15-minute online search will give you additional ideas). Just remember to keep the number of questions to a reasonable length; you don't need to show up with 5 pages of questions.

Pediatrician Background, Credentials, Experience

❑   How long have you been in practice?

❑   Are you Board Certified?

❑   Do you have any areas of subspecialty?

❑   How many doctors are in your practice?

❑   What hospitals are you affiliated with?

❑   How soon after the baby is born will you visit the baby at the hospital/birth center? Will you visit every day until we are discharged?

❑   How do you feel about parents calling during the day or after hours over "little things"?

❑   How will my after-hours call be handled?

❑   Is there a specific time during the day that you will take phone calls?

❑   Do you answer any general questions via email?

❑   Are there nurses available to answer questions during the day?

❑   Will we see you every visit, or will we see other doctors in the practice or a physician's assistant?

❑   What do you expect from me as the parent of your patient?

Office Logistics

❑   What are your office hours? Do you have any early
      morning, late evening, or weekend hours for working
      parents?

❑   How far in advance do I need to book appointments?

❑   What lab work can be performed at your office (strep
      cultures, etc.)?

❑   Who covers for you when you are on vacation?

❑   Does your office mail out reminders for scheduled
      immunizations and checkups?

Fees and Methods of Payment

❑   Do you accept our insurance?

❑   Will you bill our insurance company directly?

❑   What happens if we miss a scheduled visit? Is there a
      fee? Can we easily reschedule appointments if necessary?

Specific Concerns

❑   If you have specific concerns about breastfeeding,
      immunizations, medication, etc., be sure to address them
      with the pediatrician during your initial meeting. It is
      important that you and the pediatrician have similar care
      philosophies.

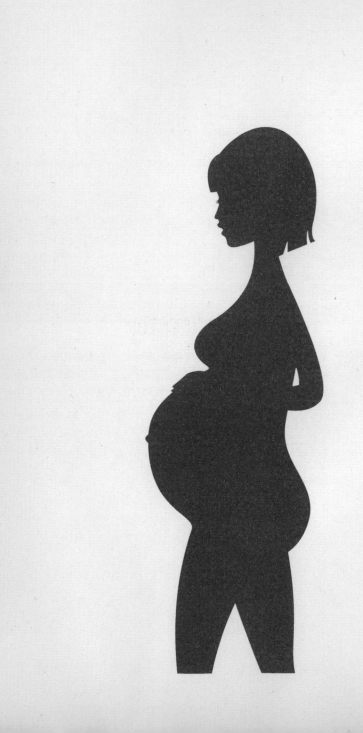

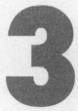

The Third Trimester

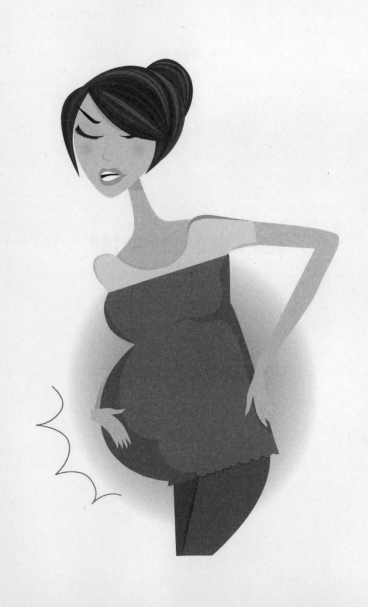

6

Preparing for Your Delivery

Whether you choose to deliver in a traditional hospital room, at a birth center, in a birthing tub, or at home, there is a significant amount of work you will need to do to prepare for what my mother always called "the watermelon through the keyhole trick!"

Childbirth Classes

Sign up for childbirth classes as soon as you can—the most popular ones fill up quickly. The best place to check first is the hospital or birth center where you will deliver, or your doctor's office. Talk to friends to find out which classes they found the most valuable before you sign up for everything you can find. Even if you plan to read all of the pregnancy books and do extensive research, there are valuable topics that will be discussed in a class. Plus, you will make friends who are due right around the same time you are!

If you sign up for a breastfeeding class, take your partner with you if at all possible. It will be very helpful for you if he is knowledgeable about breastfeeding and able to provide additional support.

Birth Plan

Before you start writing your birth plan, talk to people you trust about their birthing experiences to get the true low-down. Everyone's experience is very different, and hearing multiple stories can help you prepare for your own unique experience. It is most important to never lose sight of the fact that you will make it! All of the pain and discomfort you will face is well worth it the second you hold your little bundle of joy for the first time.

When you are writing your birth plan, remember that it is important to remain flexible; after all, your ten-page birth plan won't even make it out of your bag if the baby is breached and you have to have an emergency c-section. Be sure that your birth plan includes at least the following:

Identifying Information

❑ Due date

❑ Hospital or birth center name

❑ Doctor's name

❑ Pediatrician's name

❑ Planned delivery (vaginal vs. c-section)

Labor Preferences

❑ Others allowed in the room with you (partner, family member, doula, midwife, etc.)

❑ Preferred positions (mobile vs. stationary)

❑ Pain medication preferences

❑ Fetal monitoring preferences

Delivery Preferences

❑ Others allowed in the room with you (partner, family member, doula, midwife, etc.)

❑ Preferred delivery position

❑ Intervention preferences (vacuum, forceps, episiotomy, c-section, etc.)

Post-Delivery Preferences

❑ Whether you would like to hold or nurse the baby immediately

❑ Who will cut the umbilical cord

❑ Cord blood donation or banking preferences

Baby's Medical Treatment

❑ Who should be present for the baby's medical exam, bath, etc.

❑ Who will accompany the baby in the case that he or she is transferred to the NICU

❑ Circumcision preferences for boys

Things to Take to the Hospital

When you are packing your hospital "go bag," don't forget that after you deliver you will be roughly the same size you were at 6 months pregnant—so don't pack your skinny jeans. It takes about a week for your uterus to contract (ouch!) back to its normal size, so be patient. It is helpful to have your bag packed and ready to go a couple of weeks before your due date, just in case you deliver early and because you will not feel like doing much of anything during the last week or two of your pregnancy.

In addition to your overnight bag, it is a good idea to pack a separate labor and delivery bag with anything you will need in the delivery room. Don't forget about your partner! Chances are your partner will be spending most, if not all, of his time at the hospital with you and baby, so make sure he has a bag packed, as well.

Labor and Delivery Bag

❑   Your birth plan

❑   Pediatrician's contact information so that he/she can be notified as soon as the little one arrives.

❑   Camera (digital and video). Make sure your batteries are charged and you have the accessories you will need to download pictures (including your laptop).

❑   Music to listen to. You likely won't be able to plug in your iPod stereo, so make sure that you have plenty of batteries.

❑   Comfort items to ease your labor pain. A tennis ball inside of a tube sock is a great back massager. Raw rice inside of a tube sock can be thrown into the microwave for an instant heating pad. Your favorite scented lotion can help to ease aching muscles.

❑   Snacks for your partner and anyone else you plan to have with you during your delivery. Make sure you don't pack any of your favorite snacks in this bag, because you will likely not be able to eat while you are in labor. You wouldn't want to throw up!

❑   Phone list for calling friends and family when the little one arrives.

❑   If you are planning to donate or bank your cord blood, make sure to bring the required paperwork with you.

There are a number of additional items you will need that are provided by most hospitals. If the hospital you will be delivering at does not supply the following, you will need to bring them with you (gown, slippers, socks, extra pillows, birth ball, etc.).

Overnight Bag

❑ Nursing bra, if you plan to nurse. You'll be the most comfortable in a sleeping nursing bra or nursing camisole.

❑ Toiletries so that you can take a shower as soon as you feel ready.

❑ Pajamas. Since you will be spending the majority of your time in bed, make sure they are comfortable. Remember that you will still be roughly the size you were at six months pregnant. If you plan to nurse, make sure your top or nightgown is appropriate. If you are going to have a c-section, be sure to pack pajamas that will not irritate your incision. You may not end up wearing your own pajamas on the first day for fear that you may ruin them due to heavy bleeding, but they will come in handy on day two.

❑ Underwear. You will be given special stretchy underwear in the hospital, but you may want to pack a pair or two of your own to wear home. Be aware that you may ruin your underwear due to the heavy bleeding. Yes, they do have to be granny panties because you will be wearing a maxi pad (or two).

❑ Change of clothes for your partner, and toiletries if he will be spending the night.

❑ Going-home outfits for you and baby.

❑ Entertainment items such as a book, magazine, or movie.

❑ Your favorite snacks. Knowing that these were on hand was extra motivation for me during my labor.

Your Time in the Hospital or Birth Center

Insurance coverage and state regulations vary wildly, but one thing is certain: you will spend an extra night or two in the hospital if you have a c-section. Check with your insurance company to find out exactly how many nights you should expect to stay in the hospital. While you are in the hospital, you will be visited at least once a day by the baby's pediatrician and your doctor for quick checkups. Your nurse or a nurse's assistant will stop by regularly to check your vital signs—yes, even in the middle of the night.

While you are recovering, there will be nurses there to help you, so call them when you have questions or need assistance. The nursery is available to monitor the baby 24 hours a day if you need to get some sleep. If you are worried about an overwhelming influx of visitors, have your partner, family member, or friend manage your visitors and answer the phone for you. If you are not up for visitors, there is nothing wrong with asking people to wait until you are settled in at home to visit.

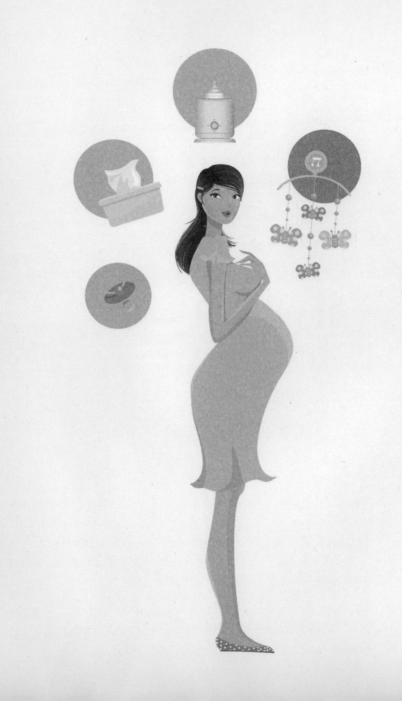

7

Preparing to Bring Your Baby Home

There is a lot of work that needs to be done around your house to get ready for the little one, that is for sure. While you can take care of all of this work after the baby comes home (or, better yet, have family and friends help), it may give you some peace of mind to have it taken care of so you don't have to do any more work when you get home. Here are the most important things to take care of.

Getting the House Ready for Baby

Laundry

❑　Wash the baby's newborn clothes so that they are ready when you get home. A newborn's skin is extremely sensitive, so make sure you use a newborn detergent like Dreft or a similar dye- and fragrance-free detergent. And do not use dryer sheets or fabric softener.

❑　Wash plenty of sheets, burp cloths, washcloths, towels, and blankets for the first week—do not underestimate how many accidents you might have!

Equipment Set-Up

❏ Get the baby's main sleeping area (bassinet, crib, Pack 'n Play, etc.) set up so that you do not have to fumble around assembling anything the day you bring baby home.

❏ Set up your diaper changing station and stock it with diapers, wipes, etc.

❏ Install the infant car seat base in your car. You will not be allowed to leave the hospital without a properly installed infant car seat. If you need help installing the infant car seat, check your local baby store, hospital, fire department, or state trooper's office for installation clinics.

Must-Have Feeding Basket

Put together a basket or small bag of the necessities you will need to have handy while you are nursing or bottle feeding the baby for 10–45 minutes every two or three hours. Yes, that is a lot of time to be glued to the couch or your glider, so make sure you have the following items within reach:

❏ Hand sanitizer

❏ Hand lotion (for your poor, overwashed hands)

❏ Water bottle (you will get very thirsty while nursing)

❏ Itzbeen, timer, or stopwatch (for timing the length of the feeding and the time between feedings)

❏ Suction bulb and infant saline nose drops (it may be easiest to suction baby's nose while he or she is eating)

❏ Burp cloth (for the inevitable spills and spit ups)

❏ Phone (to catch up on phone calls and check email)

❑   Pacifier

❑   Ibuprofen or prescription medication (for the first week or two of *your* recovery)

❑   Mylicon (to help with baby's gas)

❑   Snacks for you

Don't Forget Your Partner!

Your relationship with your partner is extremely important, and you will need each other now more than ever. You are embarking on a new adventure that can take every bit of energy and knowhow you can muster, and you will need support. You will both be very tired and at times overwhelmed, which can be a touchy combination. Do not lose sight of what brought you to this point in your relationship, and always remember that you are the baby's first example of what a relationship is—so set a good example. Try to schedule a time in the first few weeks for you and your partner to sneak out of the house for an hour or two, just the two of you. Don't underestimate how hard this might be: I cried all day thinking about going to the movies when our first son was three weeks old. I am, however, extremely glad we took the time to go on a mini-date, because it made leaving him with a sitter much easier on all of us as he got older.

Getting Ready for Your Recovery

This is the most important advice I wish I had received before the birth of my first child, because (despite my research) I was not prepared for my own recovery. It is easy to get so caught up in preparing for the baby that you forget about yourself. The discomfort and special care associated with recovering from my delivery were both more than I expected.

During your recovery, don't overdo it! The baby and your partner need you to be healthy and well rested. If you delivered vaginally and had any tearing/stitches or an episiotomy, sitting down too much can cause great discomfort. Try to lay down or stand up to relieve the pressure. If you had a c-section, sitting may also put too much pressure on your incision; so, keep your sitting time to a minimum.

Whether you have a c-section or deliver vaginally, your uterus will need to contract back to its normal size. Yes, this is as painful as it sounds. For me, the pain was somewhere in between a very bad cramp and the contractions I had while in labor. Again, something I was not prepared for. Do not be surprised if you experience the worst contractions while you are nursing— breastfeeding somehow triggers the contractions. But don't worry, this only lasts roughly a week. By the end of it, your belly will be much closer to its prepregnancy size (assuming you've cut back on the Ho Hos and Ding Dongs).

Make sure to get as much rest as you can, whenever you can! Nap when the baby is napping, accept any offers of help, and let the little things go. When friends and family come over to visit, hand them the baby and head to bed for a quick cat nap. Let's be honest, they are really only there to visit the baby!

Things to Buy

☐ Maxi pads. You can bleed or spot for up to 6 weeks postdelivery, and doctors recommend that you not use tampons. Plan accordingly!

☐ Squirt bottles for cleaning yourself while you are still too swollen or sore to wipe. You simply need to fill the bottle with warm water.

☐ Flushable wipes for when you are healed enough to wipe but are still sensitive. If you have a septic system or a history of plumbing problems, you may want to avoid flushing even flushable wipes.

❑ Place maxi pads, squirt bottle, and flushable wipes in the bathroom(s) you will use the most. A cute, decorative basket with a lid is an inexpensive and stylish way to ensure that everything is easily accessible.

❑ Granny panties, since pads will not attach to your cute little thongs. You won't want to wear thongs while you are recovering and the swelling is still going down, anyway.

❑ . Choose panties that are very comfortable and have waistlines that give. If you have a c-section, be mindful of the location of your incision: you do not want the waistline of your panties to irritate your incision.

❑ Stool Softener. Your doctor will likely prescribe stool softeners for you to take each night that you are in the hospital to decrease any discomfort. It is nice to also have this on hand when you arrive home.

❑ Thank you notes. Friends and family will likely stop by the hospital or your house with a small gift for you or the baby, so be prepared to thank them!

Meals

❑ Ensure that your pantry and freezer are stocked with plenty of no-hassle snacks and meals. Trust me, you will not feel much like cooking your first week at home.

❑ If you are fortunate enough to have friends and family who offer to cook for you, plan accordingly so that they are not all showing up on Monday evening—leaving you with too much to eat that night and nothing on tap for later in the week.

❑   Stock up on delivery and take out menus from your favorite local restaurants. While it is quick and easy to order pizza, this isn't college; and, you do need to eat a balanced diet while you are recovering, especially if you are breastfeeding!

❑   Check to see if any of your local grocery stores offer online ordering and drive-up, pick-up, or delivery ser-vices. It can be a lifesaver and well worth the small fee to not have to spend an hour at the grocery store. My local store charges $4.95 and uses my reusable grocery bags. It is well worth every penny!

Cleaning/Other Household Chores

❑   If you can fit it into the budget, hire someone to clean the house for you in the first week or two after the baby arrives. If there is no room in the budget, recruit a family member or friend who has offered to help. You can also find postpartum doulas who will help you with all of your postpartum needs.

❑   If you are particular about how laundry is washed or what cleaning products are used, be sure to make a note of your preferences and post them in the appropriate place (i.e., post laundry directions above the washer and dryer).

Childcare for Older Siblings

❑   If this is not your first child, consider having a babysitter, family member, or friend spend time with your older child or children. You are bound to be a bit sleep deprived the first couple of weeks, and your other child or children may need a little extra attention during this major change in their lives.

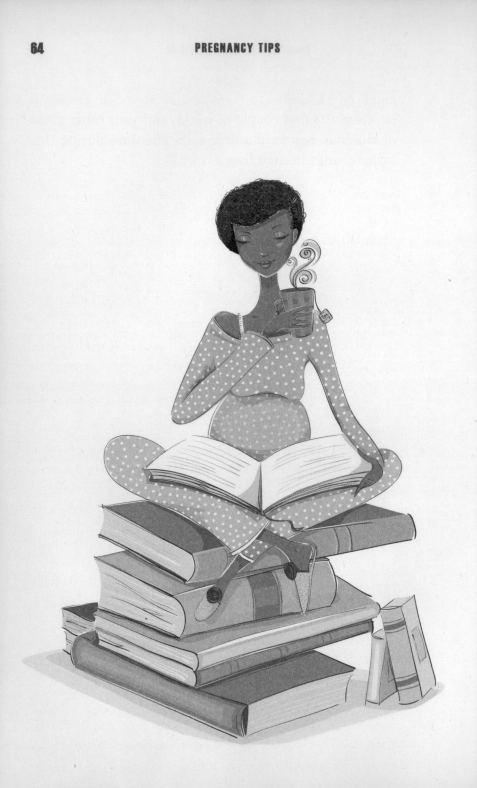

8

Reading, Reading, and More Reading

There are as many theories on how to raise a child as there are children to raise, so (don't worry!) you do not need to read all of these books. The easiest way to determine which book will be best for your new family is to talk to friends, neighbors, or family members who follow each of the different methods and see if their way of parenting is what you have in mind. Also, do not lose sight of the fact that every child is very different and may not respond to some methods. This is yet another area where you will need to remain flexible.

- *On Becoming Baby Wise,* by Gary Ezzo and Robert Bucknam. This book teaches parents how to implement a schedule and regular sleep routine.

- *The Happiest Baby on the Block,* by Harvey Karp. This book helps parents understand that the first three months are the fourth trimester.

- *Secrets of the Baby Whisperer,* by Tracy Hogg and Melinda Blau. This book helps parents understand what their babies are telling them.

❑   *The Baby Book,* by William Sears, Martha Sears, Robert Sears, and James Sears. This is a guidebook for attachment parenting.

❑   *Your Baby's First Year: Week by* Week, by Glade B. Curtis and Judith Schuler. This is a great book to guide you through each week of baby's first year.

❑   *Caring for Your Baby and Young Child: Birth to Age 5,* by The American Academy of Pediatrics. This is an extremely helpful medical reference for when something seems "off."

❑   *What to Expect the First Year,* by Heidi Eisenberg Murkoff, Arlene Eisenberg, and Sandee Hathaway. This is a follow-up book to *What to Expect When You Are Expecting,* to guide you through baby's first year.

It may be tough to find the time to fit in this additional reading on top of the pregnancy manuals, so pace yourself. The first two to three weeks of the baby's life will be a blur of feedings, diapers, and short naps. But you may be able to sneak in a chapter or two during feedings.

In order to tackle all of these baby books, my husband and I took the "divide and conquer" approach: he started *Babywise* while I started *Happiest Baby on the Block,* then we compared notes. We were able to tell within the first few chapters whether or not a parenting approach was a good fit for us. What ended up happening was that only one of us read the first few chapters of the less enjoyable book, and we both read the baby manual we preferred cover to cover.

As with all pregnancy books, these baby books will open your eyes to so many things. When I began reading *Babywise* and *Happiest Baby on the Block,* I was amazed that there are such different theories on what you should and should not do in the first month after your baby is born! Like I have said before, it is very helpful to find out what others are doing so you can make an informed decision. Don't worry, you don't have to plan your entire parenting strategy now! But you and your partner may want to decide what parenting approach you will take early on, so that you are not having this conversation at 3 A.M. while the baby is crying.

Parenting Styles

❑ Will the baby sleep in the bed with you?

❑ Will you let the baby cry it out?

❑ Will the baby use a pacifier?

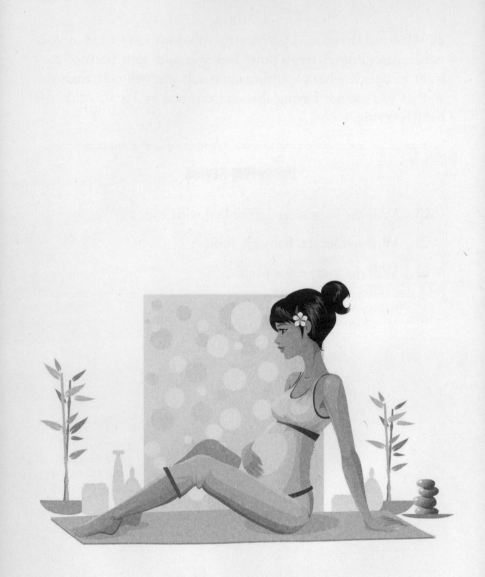

Taking Care of Yourself
and Your Partner

While you are busy preparing for the arrival of your little one and all of the craziness that will come with parenthood, do not forget to take care of yourself and your partner! Don't forget that the relationship you have with your partner is a very important one. It is very easy to get so wrapped up in your pregnancy and preparations that your relationship takes a backseat; don't let this happen. During your pregnancy, you are not the only one preparing to welcome a new life into the world. You and your partner are also preparing to become a family. Whether your baby will be entering a "traditional" family or not, you are setting an example.

Take Care of Yourself

Having a baby is one of the most wonderful and difficult things in the world, and every mother will tell you that a baby instantly becomes your number one priority. For the baby's sake, don't forget to take care of yourself. It is important to talk to your doctor before you take on any physical activity. Once you have been cleared, try to schedule some time to do something for yourself. Don't forget that time for yourself may be very limited after the baby arrives.

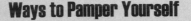

Ways to Pamper Yourself

❑   Get a prenatal massage.

❑   Spend a day at the spa by yourself or with a girlfriend.

❑   Take a day off of work for yourself.

❑   Schedule a girls' night out.

❑   Go on a date without talking about the baby.

❑   Step outside of your box: wear something funky you wouldn't normally wear.

❑   Take a prenatal yoga class.

❑   Go on a walk.

❑   Read a magazine or book that is not about pregnancy or babies.

❑   Make a list of the pregnancy "dont's" that you've been dying to do, so that you can check them off after the baby is born.

Take Care of Your Partner

Don't forget that your partner is on this wild ride with you! While you are the one with all of the aches and pains who cannot tie her own shoes, your partner has been there to listen to all of your woes and be a shoulder for you to cry on when your hormones are raging. Remember that time you spilled grape juice on your brand new top and cried for two hours straight? Perhaps you should consider doing something to thank your partner for always being there for you and helping you through the tough days.

Ways to Pamper Your Partner

❑ Surprise your partner with a little something you bought or made.

❑ Make sure your partner gets some time out with friends before the baby arrives.

❑ Surprise your partner with his favorite homemade dinner.

❑ Coordinate a surprise get together for your partner and his friends to coincide with your baby shower.

Now What?

I hope this book has saved you many hours of research and has armed you with the pregnancy tips you need to navigate through the weeks and months ahead. I also hope you feel less "clueless" about your pregnancy. With this guide at your side, you are ready to tackle everything that your pregnancy can throw your way! While there is a lot to do, just pace yourself and enjoy the experience. You'll handle it all easily!

To keep up with the latest pregnancy fashion trends, hot topics, and baby gadgets, you can follow mom bloggers and pregnancy websites. There are literally a million different blogs you can follow that contain helpful information and insights—or simply make you laugh. It is important to remember that blogs, like many things, are one person's unfiltered opinion. And you know what they say about opinions!

Pregnancy Trends and Medical Advice Sites

❑ www.thebump.com/

❑ www.fitpregnancy.com/

❑ www.babyzone.com/

❑ www.babycenter.com/

Now, go put all of your newfound knowledge to work! It is time to do a little maternity clothes shopping, buy a pregnancy medical reference book, find a prenatal yoga class, and start your registry. There's a whole lot to do before your baby arrives, but it will all come together. Just remember to relax and enjoy every minute of this wild ride.

For the latest tips and information about The Clueless Chick™, visit our website: *www.TheCluelessChick.com*. I hope you will keep coming back for more tips!

Until next time,

Jennifer

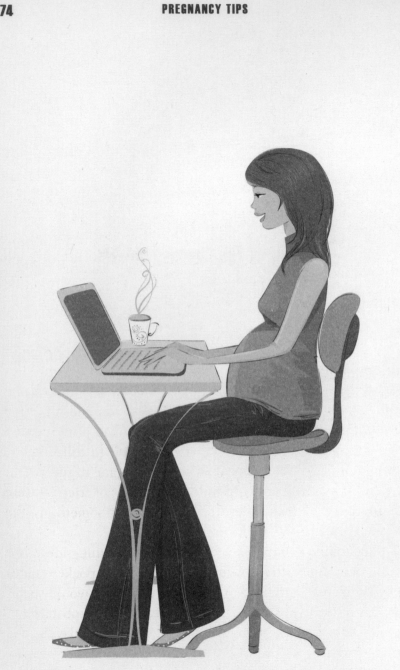

Origins of The Clueless Chick™

On June 30, 2009, my husband, Matt, and I were settling in for the night after putting our six-month-old to bed. Matt was telling me about another one of his brilliant book ideas, and I was only half paying attention. As he went on and on, it hit me that *I* needed to write a book! After all, I had just created a blog (http://www.justaskjennifer.blogspot.com) to collect all of my tips and tricks that people had been asking me to send them for years. If so many of my friends (and friends of friends) were interested in what I had to say, maybe I was on to something. The idea for The Clueless Chick™ series was born!

Matt and I immediately started brainstorming ideas and quickly determined that I would write a series of pocket guides for every woman, girlfriend, wife, and mother who would spend hours researching about all of life's milestones and obstacles if she had more than five minutes to spare in her busy day. As the quintessential Type-A/OCD overachiever, I can share all of my tips, tricks, and research to help point you in the right direction on your journey. I am here to clue you in!

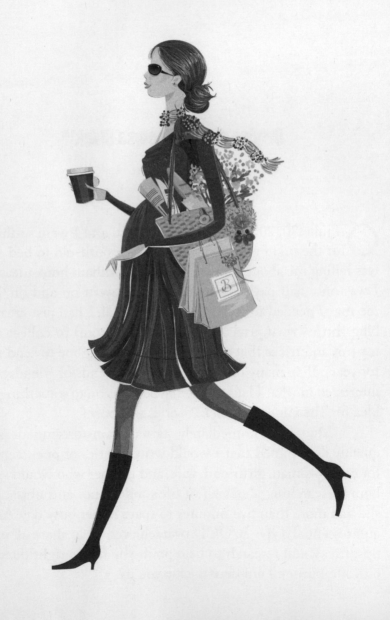

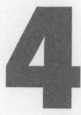

Tear It Out and

Take It with You!

Questions to Ask a Prospective Doctor

Insurance and Billing

❑ Do you accept my insurance?

❑ Will you prepare a payment plan for me?

The Practice

❑ How many doctors are in your practice? Will I meet with each doctor in your practice?

❑ How long have you been in practice?

❑ Are you board certified?

❑ Will you deliver my baby, or will it be the doctor who is on call that day?

❑ Can I speak directly to you if I have questions in between appointments?

❑ If my pregnancy is deemed "high risk," will I continue to see you, or will you refer me to another practice?

❑ Will I have to go to a lab each time blood must be drawn, or do you have a facility onsite?

❑ How frequently will I have prenatal appointments?

❑ Will there be time for me to ask questions during my appointments?

❑ Do you offer childbirth classes?

Delivery

❑ What hospitals and birth centers are you affiliated with?

❑ Will you support my birth plan and medication preferences?

❑ Will you support my decision to involve a midwife or doula in the delivery?

Questions to Ask a Day Care Provider

Cost

- ❑ How much do you charge for infant care?
- ❑ How often do your rates change?
- ❑ Do your charges decrease as the child gets older?
- ❑ What is your payment schedule (i.e., monthly, semi-monthly, or weekly)?
- ❑ What forms of payment do you accept?
- ❑ Do you charge any type of annual enrollment, materials, or other fees?
- ❑ Is there a charge to be placed on your waitlist?

Schedule and Availability

- ❑ Do you have a slot open to begin caring for my child on _____ date?
- ❑ What are your normal hours?
- ❑ Do you charge for early drop-offs or late pickups?
- ❑ Do you offer part-time slots?
- ❑ Can I drop in unannounced to visit my child?

Supplies/Materials/Food Provided

- ❑ What supplies am I responsible for, and what do you provide (diapers, wipes, bibs, etc.)?

❑ Do you provide lunch and snacks for the children?

❑ Are the meals nutritious/organic

Teachers/Care Givers

❑ What are the teachers' qualifications?

❑ What is the discipline philosophy/policy?

❑ Do you provide continuing education for your teachers or have them attend continuing education courses?

Other

❑ Do you require proof of immunizations?

❑ What safety measures do you have in place to protect my child?

❑ What is your sick child policy?

❑ Do you allow shoes to be worn in the infant room?

Baby Registry Must-Haves

Nursery Furniture

- ☐ *Crib*
- ☐ Changing table
- ☐ Dresser
- ☐ Rocker, glider, or recliner
- ☐ Bookshelves
- ☐ Nightlight (check your local home improvement store)

Nursery Miscellaneous

- ☐ Baby clothes hangers
- ☐ Baskets or organizers (for diapers, wipes, toys, etc.)
- ☐ Humidifier or vaporizer
- ☐ Diaper pail (deodorizers, bags, etc.)
- ☐ Small trash can
- ☐ Clothes hamper
- ☐ Ceiling fan (to ensure proper air circulation while the baby sleeps)
- ☐ Safety items (outlet covers, cord hiders, blind cord attachments, etc.)

Clothes

In the first couple of months you will want to dress your baby with one layer more than you are wearing, since they do not produce as much body heat.

- ❑ *Hats*
- ❑ Onesies (short-sleeved and long-sleeved)
- ❑ Pants
- ❑ *Sleepers*
- ❑ One-piece rompers
- ❑ Socks
- ❑ Hand covers (baby mittens or newborn socks)
- ❑ Seasonal clothes (light sweaters for the fall, heavy clothes for the winter)
- ❑ Swaddlers or sleep sacks
- ❑ Going-home outfit (for the trip home)

Other Linens

- ❑ *Hooded towels and washcloths*
- ❑ *Fitted crib sheets* (2–3). You will also need a waterproof liner if your crib mattress is not waterproof. It saves time and money to find a waterproof mattress for inconvenient messes.
- ❑ Crib bumper. You can get either a traditional bumper (to protect their little heads from hitting the crib slats), or a breathable bumper (to prevent them from using the bumper as a climber or getting their little faces buried in a padded bumper).
- ❑ Pack 'n Play sheet (1–2)
- ❑ Changing pad covers (2–3)
- ❑ Boppy covers (2)
- ❑ *Blankets* (for covering the infant carrier when you take the baby out in the first few weeks or for swaddling on the go)
- ❑ Bibs (for spit up and drool)

- ❑ *Burp cloths* (small and large)
- ❑ *Baby laundry detergent* (Dreft or other dye-free and fragrance-free detergent)
- ❑ Nursing cover (for nursing in public or when you have houseguests)

Travel Gear

- ❑ *Infant car seat*
- ❑ Diaper bag
- ❑ Sun shade (or two) for the car
- ❑ Extra car seat base (if the baby will be riding in more than one car)
- ❑ Backseat mirror (so you can see your little one while you are driving)
- ❑ *Stroller frame* (to snap the infant carrier into)
- ❑ Jogging stroller (for long hikes or just tooling around the neighborhood)
- ❑ Baby carrier (Baby Bjorn, ERGObaby, Moby Wrap, sling, etc.)

Play Gear

- ❑ Swing. Try to find one that plugs in so that you do not burn through batteries.
- ❑ Bouncy seat/Papasan
- ❑ Crib mobile. Make sure you get a battery-operated one that plays for 10–15 minutes. Some even have remotes.
- ❑ Play gym. Many come with a baby pillow, which is great for tummy time.
- ❑ Pack 'n Play

Miscellaneous Gear

☐   Itzbeen. This is a must-have! It keeps track of baby's last feeding, which side you last nursed on, the last diaper change, and the last nap. A timer can be set for each. There are also smartphone apps similar to the Itzbeen, such as Baby Brain and Baby ESP.

☐   Boppy (for breastfeeding)

☐   Bumbo

☐   Pacifiers and clips. Get a few different kinds to try. Make sure to get a holder that clips onto baby's clothes.

Bottle-Feeding Gear

☐   Bottles

☐   Bottle brush

☐   Bottle warmer

☐   Pitcher with lid (for making larger quantities of formula if you are exclusively bottle feeding)

☐   Dishwasher basket (for bottle parts, pacifiers, teething rings, spoons, you name it)

☐   Bottle drying rack (because you'll be washing a lot of bottles by hand)

☐   Formula

☐   Powder formula dispenser (for your diaper bag)

Health and Safety Gear

☐   Video monitor

☐   Nose bulb

☐   *Nail file/nail clippers*

☐   *Thermometer and covers*

❑　　Baby lotion. This needs to be used very sparingly on new-borns, so there is no need to stock up immediately.

❑　　Infant saline nasal drops/spray for stuffy noses

❑　　*Cotton swabs.* Safety swabs will prevent you from going too deep into the baby's ear, and regular cottonswabs are perfect for cleaning the umbilical cord stump.

❑　　*Rubbing alcohol* (for cleaning the umbilical cord)

❑　　Vasoline (if you are having a boy who will be circumcised)

❑　　Mylicon (in case the little one has gas)

❑　　Infant Tylenol

❑　　Aquaphor (great for your poor, overwashed hands)

Bathing

❑　　Infant bath

❑　　*Head-to-toe body wash*

❑　　Hairbrush

Diapering

❑　　*Diapers*

❑　　*Wipes,* wipes, and more wipes!

❑　　Diaper rash cream

❑　　Portable changing pad

Other Must-Haves

❑　　Thank you notes (for baby gifts, meals, etc.)

❑　　Camera/video camera

❑　　Baby book or scrapbook

❑　　Hand sanitizer

❑　　Antibacterial hand soap in your favorite scent

Questions to Ask a Prospective Pediatrician

Pediatrician Background, Credentials, Experience

❑ How long have you been in practice?

❑ Are you Board Certified?

❑ Do you have any areas of subspecialty?

❑ How many doctors are in your practice?

❑ What hospitals are you affiliated with?

❑ How soon after the baby is born will you visit the baby at the hospital/birth center? Will you visit every day until we are discharged?

❑ How do you feel about parents calling during the day or after hours over "little things"?

❑ How will my after-hours call be handled?

❑ Is there a specific time during the day that you will take phone calls?

❑ Do you answer any general questions via email?

❑ Are there nurses available to answer questions during the day?

❑ Will we see you every visit, or will we see other doctors in the practice or a physician's assistant?

❑ What do you expect from me as the parent of your patient?

Office Logistics

❑ What are your office hours? Do you have any early morning, late evening, or weekend hours for working parents?

❑ How far in advance do I need to book appointments?

❑ What lab work can be performed at your office (strep cultures, etc.)?

❑ Who covers for you when you are on vacation?

❑ Does your office mail out reminders for scheduled immunizations and checkups?

Fees and Methods of Payment

❑ Do you accept our insurance?

❑ Will you bill our insurance company directly?

❑ What happens if we miss a scheduled visit? Is there a fee? Can we easily reschedule appointments if necessary?

Specific Concerns

❑ If you have specific concerns about breastfeeding, immunizations, medication, etc., be sure to address them with the pediatrician during your initial meeting. It is important that you and the pediatrician have similar care philosophies.

Things to Take to the Hospital

Labor and Delivery Bag

❑   Your birth plan

❑   Pediatrician's contact information so that he/she can be notified as soon as the little one arrives.

❑   Camera (digital and video). Make sure your batteries are charged and you have the accessories you will need to download pictures (including your laptop).

❑   Music to listen to. You likely won't be able to plug in your iPod stereo, so make sure that you have plenty of batteries.

❑   Comfort items to ease your labor pain. A tennis ball inside of a tube sock is a great back massager. Raw rice inside of a tube sock can be thrown into the microwave for an instant heating pad. Your favorite scented lotion can help to ease aching muscles.

❑   Snacks for your partner and anyone else you plan to have with you during your delivery. Make sure you don't pack any of your favorite snacks in this bag, because you will likely not be able to eat while you are in labor. You wouldn't want to throw up!

❑   Phone list for calling friends and family when the little one arrives.

❑   If you are planning to donate or bank your cord blood, make sure to bring the required paperwork with you.

❑   There are a number of additional items you will need that are provided by most hospitals. If the hospital you will be delivering at does not supply the following, you will need to bring them with you (gown, slippers, socks, extra pillows, birth ball, etc.).

Overnight Bag

❑ Nursing bra, if you plan to nurse. You'll be the most comfortable in a sleeping nursing bra or nursing camisole.

❑ Toiletries so that you can take a shower as soon as you feel ready.

❑ Pajamas. Since you will be spending the majority of your time in bed, make sure they are comfortable. Remember that you will still be roughly the size you were at six months pregnant. If you plan to nurse, make sure your top or nightgown is appropriate. If you are going to have a c-section, be sure to pack pajamas that will not irritate your incision. You may not end up wearing your own pajamas on the first day for fear that you may ruin them due to heavy bleeding, but they will come in handy on day two.

❑ Underwear. You will be given special stretchy underwear in the hospital, but you may want to pack a pair or two of your own to wear home. Be aware that you may ruin your underwear due to the heavy bleeding. Yes, they do have to be granny panties because you will be wearing a maxi pad (or two).

❑ Change of clothes for your partner, and toiletries if he will be spending the night.

❑ Going-home outfits for you and baby.

❑ Entertainment items such as a book, magazine, or movie.

❑ Your favorite snacks.

Getting the House Ready for Baby

Laundry

❑   Wash the baby's newborn clothes so that they are ready when you get home. A newborn's skin is extremely sensitive, so make sure you use a newborn detergent like Dreft or a similar dye- and fragrance-free detergent. And do not use dryer sheets or fabric softener.

❑   Wash plenty of sheets, burp cloths, washcloths, towels, and blankets for the first week—do not underestimate how many accidents you might have!

Equipment Set-Up

❑   Get the baby's main sleeping area (bassinet, crib, Pack 'n Play, etc.) set up so that you do not have to fumble around assembling anything the day you bring baby home.

❑   Set up your diaper changing station and stock it with diapers, wipes, etc.

❑   Install the infant car seat base in your car. You will not be allowed to leave the hospital without a properly installed infant car seat. If you need help installing the infant car seat, check your local baby store, hospital, fire department, or state trooper's office for installation clinics.

Must-Have Feeding Basket

Put together a basket or small bag of the necessities you will need to have handy while you are nursing or bottle feeding the baby for 10–45 minutes every two or three hours. Yes, that is a lot of time to be glued to the couch or your glider, so make sure you have the following items within reach:

❑ Hand sanitizer

❑ Hand lotion (for your poor, overwashed hands)

❑ Water bottle (you will get very thirsty while nursing)

❑ Itzbeen, timer, or stopwatch (for timing the length of the feeding and the time between feedings)

❑ Suction bulb and infant saline nose drops (it may be easiest to suction baby's nose while he or she is eating)

❑ Burp cloth (for the inevitable spills and spit ups)

❑ Phone (to catch up on phone calls and check email)

❑ Pacifier

❑ Ibuprofen or prescription medication (for the first week or two of *your* recovery)

❑ Mylicon (to help with baby's gas)

❑ Snacks for you

Getting Ready for Recovery

Things to Buy

❑   Maxi pads. You can bleed or spot for up to 6 weeks postdelivery, and doctors recommend that you not use tampons. Plan accordingly!

❑   Squirt bottles for cleaning yourself while you are still too swollen or sore to wipe. You simply need to fill the bottle with warm water.

❑   Flushable wipes

❑   Granny panties

❑   Stool Softener

❑   Thank you notes. Friends and family will likely stop by the hospital or your house with a small gift for you or the baby, so be prepared to thank them!

Meals

❑   Ensure that your pantry and freezer are stocked with plenty of no-hassle snacks and meals. Trust me, you will not feel much like cooking your first week at home.

❑   If you are fortunate enough to have friends and family who offer to cook for you, plan accordingly so that they are not all showing up on Monday evening—leaving you with too much to eat that night and nothing on tap for later in the week.

❑   Stock up on delivery and take out menus from your favorite local restaurants. While it is quick and easy to order pizza, this isn't college; and, you do need to eat a balanced diet while you are recovering, especially if you are breastfeeding!

❏ Check to see if any of your local grocery stores offer online ordering and drive-up, pick-up, or delivery services. It can be a lifesaver and well worth the small fee to not have to spend an hour at the grocery store. My local store charges $4.95 and uses my reusable grocery bags. It is well worth every penny!

Cleaning/Other Household Chores

❏ If you can fit it into the budget, hire someone to clean the house for you in the first week or two after the baby arrives. If there is no room in the budget, recruit a family member or friend who has offered to help. You can also find postpartum doulas who will help you with all of your postpartum needs.

❏ If you are particular about how laundry is washed or what cleaning products are used, be sure to make a note of your preferences and post them in the appropriate place (i.e., post laundry directions above the washer and dryer).

Childcare for Older Siblings

❏ If this is not your first child, consider having a babysitter, family member, or friend spend time with your older child or children. You are bound to be a bit sleep deprived the first couple of weeks, and your other child or children may need a little extra attention during this major change in their lives.